Move.

Explore. Risk. Learn. Fail. Grow.
Act. Motivate. Dream. Design.
Create. Live. Imagine. Study.
Change. Inspire. Spark.

Achieve.

Succeed.

Age

Aging

Aging

Intelligently

Use Your Brain, Move Your Body

Dempsey Dybdahl

I don't talk to my brain
about my age.
It has no idea
how old
I am.

Introduction

I have been aging since I was born. So have you. We have that in common.

What we probably don't have in common is that I was surrounded by proactive people who aged well. They worked at it, they used all of their body all of the time to do everything, effortlessly. Active, not sedentary. They played, hiked, camped, canoed, slept well, didn't worry about tomorrow, and ate from their own garden. They were active, exuberant, fearless.

My vision was to be just like them: wholly alive until the day I drop dead. No dementia, no debilitating illness, no slowing down. That's my choice. Your decision depends on you. But there's a cost.

We had conversations about the value of sleep for stress relief, of eating right to feed the brain for learning, of biking instead of taking the bus, of being always active, always engaged. This, when I was young.

I learned the secret of aging well by being around people who did it well. I continue their legacy.

And, I hear that I am aging well, Aging Intelligently. But then, I had good training.

Contents

If willpower worked, we wouldn't need self-help and diet books

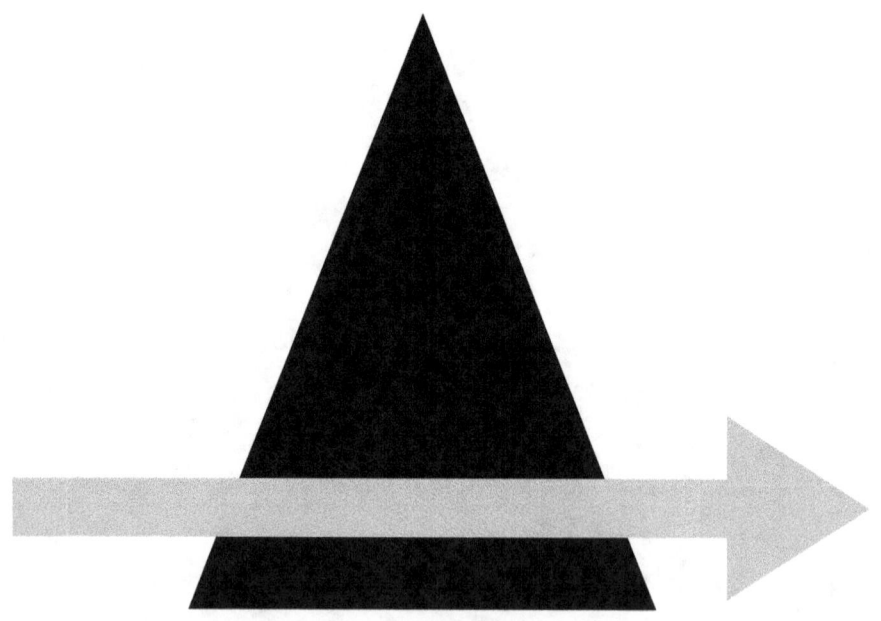

Problem

Are You Still Looking Good As You Age?

We know that stress makes us look old. Decrease the stress in our lives (good luck) and our skin improves. Yes, yes, yes…..we already know that.

Think about managing stress, not eliminating it. Management is a good coping skill; it just takes practice. Avoidance is a bad coping skill, at which we are much too good. Stress is everywhere and we need a certain amount to function. The stress of waiting for Christmas is much different than the stress of waiting for your father to arrive home to view your not-so-stellar report card. A haggard, fearful face does not present well to a father expecting better grades.

But stress is not the only thing that makes us look old. Antidepressants age our skin, as does smoking (duh) and sun exposure. Case Western Reserve University, in Cleveland, did a study on facial photographs of identical twins. They wanted to know who looked older, and why. What they discovered is that stress, depression, smoking, and sun exposure make us seem older than we are. Who wants that?
It's up to each of us how we look: wrinkled, craggy, weathered, run over, toughened, used up.

Or: radiant, stunning, fabulous, kind, fresh, open, active.

I don't mind my age. I certainly do not want to appear older than I am, and I don't mind anyone thinking that I am younger than I am. It isn't that I am vain, which I am; it is that I want to look as good as I can for as long as I can. And function just as well. They go hand in hand.

The only person who goes to Arizona in July and doesn't go in the sun is me. I know about sun and wrinkles. I don't need a tan; I just want to be warm. Smoking is something I never took up, and that leaves stress (eek!) and depression (groan). Managing both is a skill and a process on which I am working, and by being less stressed and combating depression, I move with more freedom and I am more active. And oh yes! I look better.

Age like you mean it

WILLPOWER

IS LIKE ANY OTHER MUSCLE;

IT NEEDS DAILY EXERCISE

TO STAY IN SHAPE

How Many Things Do You Do At Once?

My mother had an odd habit: she would turn down the radio in the car when she felt lost, so she could think. I thought it was weird. In the house, when she was trying to concentrate on, say, a new recipe, she would turn off the music until she had all the ingredients assembled. It turns out that she really wasn't nuts. It was her brain on overload. Too much information, not enough processing skill. But thinking is a skill, like everything else. If we work at it, we get better. If we don't, well...turn down the radio.

Neuroscience once again explains this odd behavior. By now, most of us know that multi-tasking doesn't work. You can go back and forth between two tasks, but doing two things at the same time diminishes both. It's harder, and takes longer, which defeats the purpose of trying to get more done in a shorter amount of time. It is quicker to prioritize the work that needs to be done, then accomplish it one task at a time. According to Steven Yantis, a professor at Johns Hopkins University, listening, say, on a cell phone and driving at the same time has a cost. Driving suffers. Another example that cell phones and driving don't mix. Like we need more reminders.

It is also more difficult to think at all, much less multi-task when you are tired or depressed. Your brain just isn't functioning. It needs fuel and activation, and maybe some rest.

We have a need to do more, with less time. It's nuts! Sometimes slowing down speeds you up, because you can concentrate on one thing at a time, giving it your full attention, then moving on to one more thing. That way, you don't feel overwhelmed during the day and frazzled at the end of it. You feel good about what you did, leaving you refreshed to do it again tomorrow, instead of dreading a repeat of the frustration of today.

Accomplishing tasks to "almost done, but not really" has another cost as well: stress. And by now you know, if I have harped enough about this, stress ages us prematurely, and shortens our lives. I don't care how cool it is, smoking a cigarette, yakking on your cell phone, eating lunch (because you are running late), and driving all at the same time is not a good idea.

By working on tasks one at a time, you get better at each task, and accomplish more. It's one less stress.

Dempsey Dybdahl

no

unnecessary

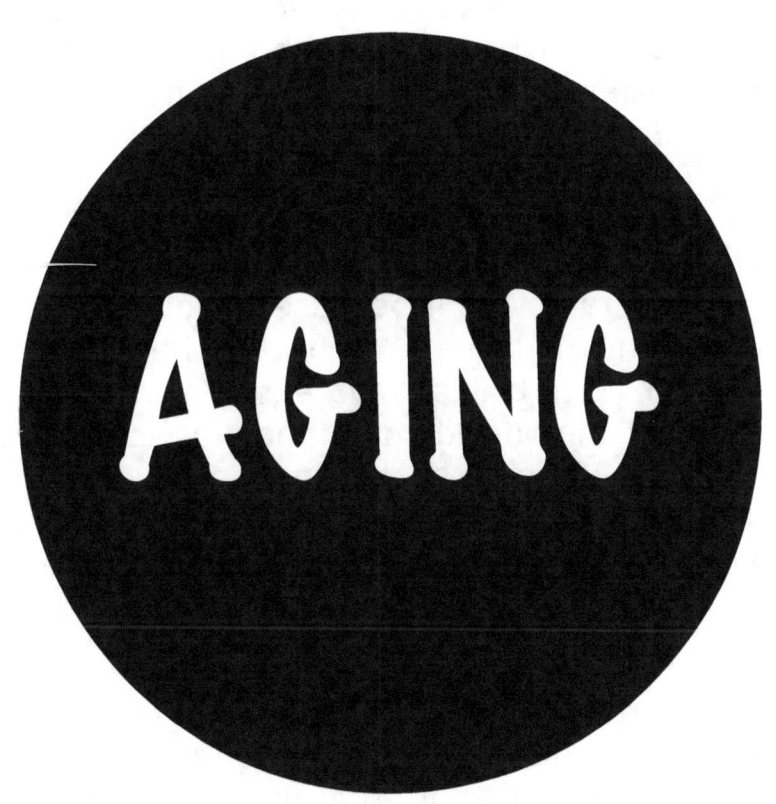

What's a Senior, and Who Decided that Definition?

I take issue with the word "senior". As in, I am a senior. Senior what? Senior to whom? I am 65. I hardly think of myself as a senior, citizen or otherwise.

Most of the dictionaries that I consulted defined senior as being senior (or older) to someone else, or a senior (versus a sophomore) in high school, or a person with a higher standing or rank (a Senior fellow of a college), or Senior and Junior (father and son). So how did we get to an older adult becoming a senior citizen? What? Senior to younger adults? And how did it get such a bad rap? Was it because of Social Security and Medicare? You have to be 60, 62, 65, 67, or 70 to collect payment. What's up with that? Can't they decide on an age for seniors? If a person is 70 and a senior, then is the person 67 not senior? Because you have to be senior to someone. So is an 11 year old a senior citizen to a 5 year old?

We add attributes to senior citizens, like infirmity, lacking mobility, slowing down, and pathetic balance without realizing the injustice that we have done to older individuals who still are vibrant, move well, stay strong. Some 12 year olds can't balance, and fall down a lot. Are they having a senior moment?

I think we should do away with the designation of seniors as a group of people. The French have the right idea. Older adults are men and women of "a certain age". That sounds more uplifting and positive than "senior citizen".

A "person of a certain age" sounds like they can still move. A senior citizen? Not so much.

Think of aging intelligently as your new job.

Consider

everything

an

experiment

Not The Same Old Age

Maybe you're thinking that you can keep on doing the same old thing, and it won't matter. Sometimes you eat the wrong foods, maybe too much food. Sometimes you drink a little more than you should, don't feel so great the next morning. What the heck! You get over it. Maybe you don't drink or eat so much the next time. You still see yourself as that strong and vibrant 27-year-old, on top of the world, tiger by the tail, blah, blah, blah.

And working out? Well............maybe not as much as you used to, but still, you fit in time when you can. You still run a couple of times a week, or bike, or go to the gym, but not always. Work, sometimes, is pressing, your boss wants you to stay late, the kids have school activities, your spouse has plans. Things happen, and after all, you ARE getting older and slowing down. It's the aging process.

On the other hand, maybe you are buying the Kool-Aid that says that aging=slowing down, not so mobile, knees hurt, lower back is a problem, eyes aren't so good. All because you're aging.

Kill me now if I ever believe that. Because, you see, belief is part of the problem. Or the solution. What you believe is what you support. If you believe that you cannot play basketball anymore, your body responds to that. Your brain will support whatever you believe. Aging becomes the list of can't: I can't play tennis, I can't run anymore, hiking hurts my knees and ankles, I am afraid that I will fall off my bicycle and hurt myself, downhill skiing is downright scary.

You choose that belief. Your brain will believe and support anything you tell it. By supporting your fears about aging, you in fact age quicker.

Do you realize that you talk to yourself all the time?

What are you saying?

Try saying something different. Try moving more to stay in shape. Move everything: neck, spine, hips, ankles, feet, hands. All that movement, that joint mobility, sends signals to your brain, assuring your brain that you are safe, that this maneuver is a teeny bit scary but still manageable on a small scale, that age is a product of what you tell your brain.

Tell your brain something intelligent: that you still have a lot to offer the world, that you can still move well. Go kick someone's butt!

Go out there in the real world and start using your brain and your talents, challenging yourself mentally and physically, every day until the day you die.

If someone paid you to age better, you would.

yak, yak, yak

blah
blah
blah

Dempsey Dybdahl

Price

Knowing

is not enough;

we must apply.

Willing

is not enough;

we must do.

Johann von Goethe

Dempsey Dybdahl

Nothing is ever accomplished by a reasonable man

American proverb

Dempsey Dybdahl

You Have To Pay

Few of us age gracefully, gently, hair-color-even and wrinkle free. Most of us have to exert some effort, and some money.

I bet that Sophia Loren doesn't look that stunning first thing in the morning. On the other hand, I bet she doesn't look that bad either.

Still............

You have to work at it and pay to look good into old age. Get over thinking that it's going to be cheap, and that you can keep on doing the same old thing that you have always done.

You can't.

It is going to take more effort. Your body doesn't function the same way it did one hundred years ago, when you were so much younger. But it isn't impossible. You don't have to give up. It isn't hopeless.

Start now, today, making better choices.
Continue every day until the day you drop dead.
You get no more free days of abusing your body

with little sleep, too much drugs and drink, plates of fried food, bad attitude, and draining relationships. Now you have to pay attention to how you feel each day, and how well you function. If you don't like how you function, do something different. Go for a walk, get more sleep, drink more water, rid yourself of toxic relationships, eat more fruits and vegetables. Start small, start often, start over. It's a decision that you pay for with the kind of life you choose by your actions.

Be the person you were meant to be.

Never love anybody who treats you like you are ordinary.

Oscar Wilde

IN THE *L O N G* RUN,

WE **SHAPE** OURSELVES.

THE *PROCESS* NEVER

ENDS **UNTIL** WE DIE.

AND THE CHOICES

WE MAKE ARE OUR OWN

RESPONSIBILITY

Eleanor Roosevelt

Deliberate Practice

Vladimir Horowitz was approached by a piano student who gushed, " I would give my life to play as well as you". To which Horowitz replied, "I did".

It's about taking the time to practice with the express intention of getting better. It isn't just banging on the piano keys for an hour while the timer runs out, it isn't about practicing during commercials on TV, it isn't about playing as fast as you can through all your material so you can say you practiced. It's about actually paying attention, going slowly, correcting errors at the time of the error, concentrating on each movement, paying attention to your posture, remembering to breathe, and relaxing while you play. Playing piano should be fun, not the drudgery your mother thought up for you when you were 10 years old and precocious. You should enjoy yourself, feel lighter afterwards, and energized. Otherwise, quit now and stop torturing yourself.

Piano is not the only victim of inattention. We do most things by rote, and therefore, our brain retains little, if any, of what we learn. We can be so much better than we are, just by demanding more of ourselves.

Pay attention to becoming a better employee, spouse, parent, friend. Deliberate practice works on relationships, as well as piano, tennis, hiking, and beating your neighbor at ping pong. Deliberate practice is an attitude requiring focus, concentration, and commitment. If you want to get better, practice with intent. If you don't care, then don't expect great results. I play pool, and I am terrible at it. But I don't care. I play for the comic relief of everyone else. I also work at being flexible and strong, and I am good at that. I pay attention there, because it matters. I don't pay attention to pool, because, well, who cares?

Pick your battles in life. The ones that are important, treat with respect. That's how you get good. If it matters.

We don't stop playing games

because we grow old;

we grow old because

we stop playing games.

George Bernard Shaw

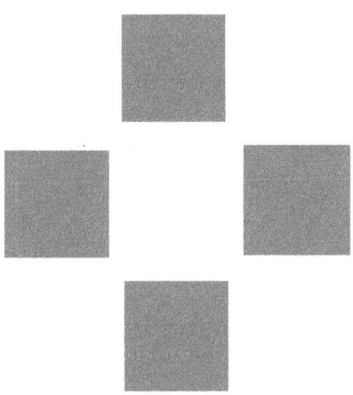

Dempsey Dybdahl

HOW OLD WOULD YOU BE

IF YOU DIDN'T KNOW
HOW OLD YOU ARE?

SATCHEL PAIGE

No Pain, No Gain

The theory of no pain, no gain is ignorant. I can't make it any clearer, and yet, a lot of us grew up with that theory, and still subscribe to it. "Work it until it hurts, feel the burn, then do 2 more repetitions." Does that sound familiar? Indeed. Most athletics was built on no pain, no gain. "They" (whoever they are, at the moment) say that you are weak, mentally soft, and you need more conditioning. You need to work through the pain you are experiencing to get stronger. Just buck up!

But it's wrong, and here's why: neuroscience. Pain is your brain and your nervous system talking to your body, trying to get you to stop or make a change in what you are currently doing, or a position you are in, or a load on a particular part of your body.

If you move concrete blocks to make a fence in your yard, and your back hurts, do you generally stop moving the blocks around? Not usually. Because you need to get the fence finished. You take Advil, telling yourself that the pain isn't so bad (it is!) and it's normal to hurt after moving concrete blocks. It isn't, if you listen to your body. Start listening to what your brain is screaming at you, and figure out how to respond without stupidity involved.

The next time you feel pain, STOP. Get help, slow down, change your position to lessen the load, but for heaven's sake, do not continue doing whatever it is that is causing the pain. It will only get worse. It never gets better. Your brain will escalate the pain until you can no longer move for an extended period of time, maybe forever if you continue to ignore it.

Living pain free is normal.

It's never too late to be who you might have been.

George Eliot

Dempsey Dybdahl

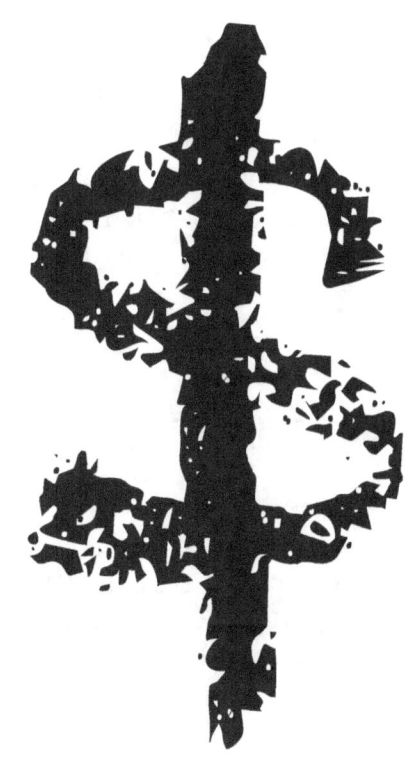

how much?

Smart Aging Is Work: How Much Does It Cost?

What got you here in life is not going to get you to the end of your life. You have less time; you need to move faster, do more. There are no more free rides; your youth will not save you. You are going to have to work a lot smarter just to maintain. Which means, you need to be more creative. And efficient.

You can still be active, agile, outrageous, opinionated with substance, intelligent, fearless, and fun. But it will cost you more time, maybe more money. You might need a trainer to keep you on track. If you want to age intelligently, that's a price you will pay. Think about on what you spend your money: dining out, good wine, your appearance to yourself and others, your kids or your pets, travel, education. Education? Getting older is about getting educated about getting older. You need to know how to fight gravity, how often and which parts of your body to keep moving, how to combat that spare tire around your middle, what foods might affect you diet-wise, how little sleep you can tolerate and still function efficiently. These are not things you thought about before. This is new.

Dempsey Dybdahl

In youth, a lot of us could function on coffee, skipping breakfast, 2 hours of sleep, too much work in not enough time, and bad relationships. None of it much mattered, because we were young and invincible. Jobs might come and go: one year I had 14 W2 forms at tax time. Ok, they were all for bartending and cocktail waitressing, and it is a flaky business, but still, that's a lot of jobs. I had no health insurance, no health issues, no weight problem, no savings, no worries, no fear, 6 roommates and a car payment of $65 a month. I was on top of the world. I was young.

Things change, time accelerates. Christmas used to take forever to arrive. Now, it's here way too soon.

Now I find that eye drills are useful while waiting for the light to change. Abdominal exercises help pass the time in bumper to bumper traffic. Standing when having a phone conversation is good, and I try to walk when having an in-person conversation.

I didn't use to do any of this, but then, I used to be invincible. I like feeling sorta, kinda, somewhat invincible as I age. I don't want to feel like I can no longer do the things that make me happy, so I am willing to do the work necessary to be able to have choice in life. I still like to do cartwheels. I don't want to stop because of my age. So I do the work. Aging intelligently takes focus and deliberate, consistent practice. It doesn't seem like work if I still have choice. And choice in life....is everything.

Act as if what you do makes a difference.

It does.

William James

Dempsey Dybdahl

Thoughts

The secret of aging intelligently

is found

in your daily routine

Good Health is the Absence of Disease

This is common sense. Think about it. There is no other way to describe good health, other than lack or absence of disease.

Most people would not say that they have a disease, but some synonyms that they would use include ailment, complaint, complication, disorder, illness, infirmity, sickness, trouble. It's all the same thing: disease, any condition that includes dysfunction of the body, distress, or social problems. For instance, Tourette Syndrome is a neurological disorder and a social disease. It causes involuntary movements, and vocalizations called tics (the social disease part). Science points to abnormalities in certain brain regions including the basal ganglia, frontal lobes, and cortex. These in turn have issue with the circuits that interconnect these areas and the neurotransmitters responsible for communication along the nerves.

It affects dopamine, serotonin, and norepinephrine, which our brain needs to function effectively.

What does it really mean? Our body isn't talking to itself very well. The signals along the nerve paths are not firing. If our brain isn't working correctly, we have less than optimal function throughout the rest of our body. We pay a price for this in balance, visual skills, and mobility. We have disease. Don't wait until it's cancer or stroke or something big to start thinking about brain health. Start today.

Poor brain health can be helped with exercises that stimulate the brain: crossword puzzles, playing an instrument, learning a new language or anything else, coordination drills, joining the Roller Derby. Anything novel and new can stimulate the brain to create better neural paths, better communication. This is why lifelong learners and fearless adventurers fare better than people who are not.

It all gets back to keeping disease in check before it gets carried away with itself. Keep learning, get enough sleep, eat with intent instead of boredom, move more. It all matters.

I sit down to work each morning

at 9am,

and the muse

has learned to be on time.

Pyotr Ilyich Tchaikovsky

Think Of Yourself As An Athlete

Joe Montana was an football athlete. Michael Jordan, basketball. Gordon Ramsey is still a chef athlete. And you are an athlete. Maybe not a professional one, but still, an athlete. And here's why, according to the Merriam-Webster dictionary: an athlete is a person skilled or trained in exercises, sports, or games involving strength, coordination, and speed.

A mom who lugs two sacks of heavy groceries up three flights of stairs is an athlete. It is an exercise involving strength and balance. A husband who pushes his wife in a wheelchair has arm strength. A dad who coaches his kid's soccer team runs up and down the field. They are all athletes.

If we have established that you are acting like an athlete, then start thinking like one. It will change your concept of yourself, in a good way. An athlete moves. He, or she, concentrates on the physical demands needed and produces skill, strength and agility, whether it's backing into a tight parking spot, gardening for three hours, or walking the dog.

An athlete is active. A sedentary person is not. Sedentary people sit more than they stand, they slump with rounded shoulders and a forward head position, and sleeping is their best activity.

Are you active, or sedentary?

Being an athlete is a mind set. We determine how we see ourselves. We talk to ourselves all the time. What are we saying? Are we active, able to do whatever we choose, not afraid of jumping and hurting our ankles or knees? An active person sporadically takes the stairs instead of the elevator, occasionally walks instead of drives, doesn't need a chair to wait in line for the rock concert tickets. They are used to standing and moving around. Because they see themselves as active, not sedentary. An active person is a moving person and an athlete, and still has choices in life. Statistics say that active people live longer than sedentary people. Let's start moving more.

The **curious**

are

never

bored...bored...bored...bored

bored...bored...bored...bored

bored...bored...bored...bored

Solution

You age how you act,

not how you feel.

Some days you feel awful.

If you act like you feel great,

you will,

sooner than you think.

My Back Pain Needs A Better Dialog

Pain is the body talking to the brain, and the most pain receptors live in and around the lumbar spine. Which might explain why, as you age, you seem to have more low back pain.

It isn't because you are aging; it's because you are not moving.

Years of sedentary lifestyle, lack of exercise, and poor posture take their toll. The spine compresses, bad habits form from disuse or accumulative injury, and low grade back pain becomes a persistent reality. It isn't there all the time, but it appears when we're stressed: we don't get enough sleep, work is driving our lives, food choices are less than stellar, and Aunt Ethel comes to visit. All that stress goes somewhere. It goes to where there are an excess of nociceptors: pain receptors. It shoots to the low back. Oweeeeee!

Why there?

The spinal cord is protected in a sheath by the spinal column. Around the lumbar spine (low back), the spinal cord exits that protective sheath. The nerves travel through the hips and down the legs. By walking, we stimulate the nerves that run through our legs back into our hips and spine. We provide our own protection for our nervous system. Nerves that can move are happy nerves. Happy nerves allow the body to move with ease.

The next time you encounter low back pain, do not sit down and be still, hoping the pain will go away. It probably will not.

Instead, go for a walk, even if it's only around your work space or house. Move your entire spine gently. Bend forward and sideward, as long as it doesn't hurt. If it does, slow down, make the motions smaller, or stop. Rotate your head from side to side, and ear to shoulder. Open and close your mouth as wide as you can, to move your jaw. Move it sideways as well.

The top of your spine talks to the bottom of your spine, which is where that low back pain lives. By having a kinder, gentler approach to moving pain free, you help yourself overall, and maybe that pain lessens or goes away. It's you being responsible for you. Long healthy life is not a gift; you have to work for it.

Aging is something you do,

not something you are.

One is an active verb;

one is a passive noun.

Are you active or passive?

Can You Change Your Posture With Your Shoes?

We don't spend a lot of time thinking about shoes, other than as a fashion statement or in terms of an activity. We have running shoes, hiking boots, high heels, boating shoes, flip flops. We primarily wear shoes to protect our feet from sharp objects on the ground and dropped bags of groceries from above. We don't think about what the shoe does to our feet.

Humans were not born wearing shoes. Nor were they born with car keys in their hands, but very few 16 year olds understand that. Shoes have a purpose, and several things can interfere with that purpose. Heels, for instance. Does anyone really think that 3 inch high heels are good for your feet? Yes I know they make your legs look great, and you appear taller and thinner. The bad news is, they alter the natural erect state of the body column. In other words, your posture is now out of alignment. All your weight is on the balls of your feet, meaning your feet are less stable. The hips are no longer in line with the spine, which is no longer in line with the head. Because of instability, there exists tension in the body that wasn't there before, and tension (stress) kicks up cortisol, which adds to weight gain. Oh wait, if you take up smoking to combat weight gain……….

If the shoe does not flex forward to backward, it creates inflexibility where the ball of the foot attaches to the toes. That walking gait you have when you are barefoot is now restricted. If the toe of the shoe contains a slight incline up (like many sneaker-type shoes), it causes metatarsal stress symptoms. The toes do not relax. If you spend all day in shoes that do not allow your toes to relax, they will have trouble relaxing when you remove your shoes. It creates a bad habit for your feet. Toes need to relax with the rest of the body.

Finally, if the shoes do not flex forward, backward, and sideways, the tactile sensory nerve endings in your feet cannot feel the floor through the shoes. The shoe forces your foot to move as a whole, not as individual bones working together. But your foot isn't a whole. It has 26 bones that need to move to give you a sense of sure-footed walking. Your brain has no sense of how stable your footing is on the floor. That is also added stress to the body, and there's that cortisol response again.

I know that certain situations demand steel toes and other specific minded footwear. I have high heels that I occasionally wear. When I return home, I kick off my shoes, rub my feet, and move my feet as much as possible. I go barefoot as much as I can so I do not have to be dependent on shoes for support. My own feet can support me, if I give them a chance.

We were born barefoot. Being tactile with the ground grounds us, and improves our posture. People with better posture live longer.

Breathe before you answer a question. Less stupid comments will come out of your mouth.

There is a battle of two wolves inside us all. One is evil. It is anger, jealousy, greed, resentment, lies, inferiority and ego. The other is good. It is joy, peace, love, hope, humility, kindness, empathy, and truth.

The wolf that wins? The one you feed.

Cherokee proverb

Today's Brain Lesson: Amygdala, Hippocampus, and Exercise

Living in the most protected area of our brain, the amygdala is our fear and emotion center. That lizard brain wants to protect us when we feel threatened. A cheetah may be chasing us, or a ride at Disneyland, the State Fair, or Wild Water Waves may be too scary. Driving at night is fearful for some people, and approaching our car in an underground parking structure when no one else is around can be equally nerve wracking. It's all fear, and the signals come from the amygdala, the nervous nelly of our body that lives in our brain.

The hippocampus, also in our brain, stores long term memory. It is believed that Alzheimer's begins in the hippocampus, then spreads outward to other parts of the brain. No one is sure how or why it starts.

Ok, brain lesson is over. And why should anyone care?

What we are beginning to see is that exercise lowers stress, which reduces fear, and impacts

memory. That's how all three are related:
exercise, the amygdala, and the hippocampus.

We actively change our brain through our
impulse signals to the amygdala and
hippocampus, by exercising, which determines
how we see, and react to, the world. And, of
course, how we age. Exercise can literally save
our life. Any exercise: walking, running,
swimming, jumping; you get the picture.

You don't have to like exercise, but then do you
like dementia?

Think how smart you will sound when you throw
words around like amygdala and hippocampus.
Because exercise also makes you smarter. That
certainly beats dementia.

Try walking 30 minutes a day, not leisurely.
Actively. Like you want to get somewhere. How
many times can you sit down in a chair and
stand up in a minute? Take your bicycle out of
the closet, throw the laundry off of it, and go for
a ride. Pretend you are a Rockette, and kick your
legs in the air. Can you kick for 2 minutes? How
about 4?

It isn't hard to start moving, and then it isn't hard to keep doing it. You just have to start. Take one step, then another. Then watch out for the cascade.

It takes about ten years to get used to how old you are.

stress

stress

Stress

stress

stress

Travel somewhere you have never traveled before, and do something that you have not previously done. And do it this year.

Oh Glorious Sleep...

Not everyone, but most of us need about 8 hours of sleep. Sadly, we get by on 6 1/2 hours, and it isn't uncommon to survive on 5 hours of sleep. For most of us, that's what we are doing with 5 hours of sleep: surviving. Barely. Not thriving, not growing, not thinking clearly, not focusing. We are surviving, and not well at that.

Think about how you feel the day after you haven't slept well: groggy and annoyed. Lack of sleep leads to poor memory, increased impulsiveness, and poor judgement. To say nothing of crankiness. You don't think, you make stupid decisions, then blame someone else.

Following a bad night's sleep, our overwhelming thought is how tired we are. In an effort to function, we might drink more rocket fuel coffee, and shove a quick, fat-laden breakfast down our throats. Which brings up weight gain and lack of sleep. Oh yes, there's a correlation. Our system releases more ghrelin, a hormone produced by the cells lining the stomach that stimulates appetite. Ergo, we think that we are hungry, so we eat more. Ghrelin appears to make high-calorie foods look more appealing. Ghrelin loves donuts. This stresses the body, and stress, plus loss of memory, leads to suppressed immunity. We become sick more often. Stress throws glucose and cortisol into blood circulation, which eventually produces diabetes. It adds to cardio-vascular disease. Oh, the things that will happen when you go without sleep....

Sleep increases concentration, attention, decision making, creativity, social skills and health. It extends your quality of life.

Sleep decreases mood change, stress, anger, impulsiveness, drinking and smoking. It limits poor choices.

In cases of mental illness, there is often sleep disruption, creating a loop back to the mental illness.

Sleep is a skill that needs to be practiced well and consciously, like anything else. To encourage deep, sustained sleep, darken the room and keep it cool, dim the lights before bedtime, and stop eating a couple of hours before retiring. Do yourself and everyone else a favor. Get some sleep.

U

O

The illiterate of the future are
not those who can't read or
write, but those who cannot
learn, unlearn, and relearn.

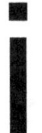Alvin Toffler

E

i

How Moving the Eyes Affects Aging

We talk to ourselves all the time. What are we saying? I'm too old; I feel foolish doing something unfamiliar; that ride is too scary, what if I get hurt? It's too much effort and I'm retired. I should have started years ago, now it's too late.
Your body talks back to you through pain, stiffness, less range of motion, fatigue.
This is the dialog we have with ourselves.

Thoughts, beliefs, and actions. What we think, our cultural beliefs, and how we move controls our aging process. We are afraid of the "O" word: old.

If you don't change anything, be prepared to age badly. Look for the rocking chair and the nice retirement home now. Be prepared when the time comes.

As we age, our balance gets worse. It isn't because of aging. It's because of not moving. If we improve our balance, we are less fearful of moving. It's just practice, over and over and over.
Try this: walk across a room with your eyes open. Easy peasy, yes? Try the same thing with your eyes closed. The difference? Your eyes help

you move better. About 70% of how we move comes from our visual system: what we see and how our brain interprets it.
If we improve our visual system, we improve our balance.

The visual system (your eyes) and the vestibular system (your balance) and the proprioceptive system (movement) talk to each other. Or they should. If you move your eyes more, your balance improves, and you move easier.

When balance improves, we feel stable, which reduces fear, which leads to more moving, which leads to longer life. By exercising eye muscles, night vision improves, and we exhibit less fear of driving at night. With improved balance, we don't drape on the handrail going down stairs. We feel sure of foot placement. We might even let go of the handrail.

This is the dialog between you and your body. When you move more, practice balance by moving your eyes more, you have less pain, less stiffness, more confidence, less fatigue. You can have a dialog with your body and it doesn't argue with you.

Use your eyes more, outside their normal range, to improve your balance.

Try this: practice eye circles as big and smooth as you can. Slow down, make the circles fluid, not jumpy. Keep them smooth. Standing may make you feel unsteady, so sit until you get good at it. Do 6-8 circles one way, then reverse. Breathe. You may feel some eye strain; it's your extra ocular eye muscles beginning to work again, after a long rest, maybe years.
Repeating this drill every day will improve your vision, improving your balance, improving your confidence in moving. You might move more. You might live longer.

If someone paid you to move, you would move more.

While we don't always get what we want,

we always get what we choose.

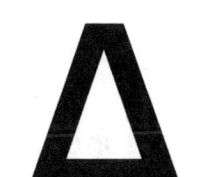

A

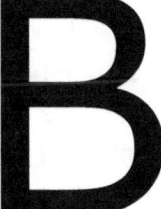

B

Aging and The Lymph System

Aging is a choice that we make everyday. We wake up and choose to age by what we do and what we think. If we want to age better, and more intelligently, we need to move more.

When your body doesn't move, it becomes sluggish. Systems slow down. Think about slouching on a sofa watching television, or sitting at a computer all day. Lymph fluid doesn't move along the accumulation of waste: parasites, viruses, toxins, infection, old dead cells. One of the ways that the lymph nodes and liver get rid of waste is through respiration, as well as the skin (perspiration), the kidneys and colon. But the lymph system needs muscle contraction to move along waste. There are no valves and pumps, like the heart. The lymph system relies on movement to keep it running efficiently. By not moving, the lungs don't expand and contract fully.

Why do we care about something very little of us know anything about? The lymph removes waste from the body, and that's a big deal. The longer waste sits in the body, the more damage it can do. Blood carries nutrients and oxygen to our cells, lymph fluid removes waste residue. Think of it as the waste water sewer system, the metabolic garbage can of the body, the oil that keeps the engine running.

The lymph system consists of the spleen, thymus, tonsils, plus the lymph nodes, fluid, and vessels. It is four times larger than the blood system, probably because of all the waste that has to be moved and ultimately removed. What? You thought you had no waste? Cells regenerate all the time; the old dead cells have to go somewhere.

Signs that you may have a lymph issue include swelling or edema (think long plane trips), psoriasis, chronic fatigue, constipation, arthritis, and clogged skin pores. That could include acne. Too much waste creates a lymph backup. The immune system weakens, and this is not good news. Performance and daily functioning are compromised. And your brain fogs because your waste system is clogged. Makes more sense now?

So...here's a thought: laugh more, breathe deeply, jump up and down and act crazy. The life you are saving is yours. And it will slow the aging process by keeping everything tip top and running smoothly. Even if I am wrong, and I am not, what do you lose by moving more in your life?

Life is change.

Growth is optional.

Choose wisely.

Dempsey Dybdahl

More Thoughts

Some cause happiness

wherever they go;

others,

whenever they go.

Oscar Wilde

Are You Sitting On Your Asset?

On average, we sit for nine hours a day. We sit while reading, eating, driving, working on the computer, yakking on the phone, watching television, writing. We sit an amazing amount of time, nine hours, while we are awake. The rest of the time we lay down. We sit more than we sleep. We are sedentary people in this country, and overweight. That statistic isn't getting any better.

What to do?

Stand up. One of the easiest things we can do to change this repetitive pattern of bad behavior leading to weight issues is to stand. Stand up to talk on the phone, or watch television. I have seen standing platforms for people who work at desks, with treadmills attached.

Standing burns calories. It tones the body. Sitting relaxes everything by taking the tension out of muscles. The body compresses, sinks into itself and becomes small. The joints get stiff, especially in the spine, the neck, and feet. You become a slug. A body at rest.......stays there. It takes inertia to move a body so rested.

It's habit forming to rest all the time. No one needs that much rest. Maintenance mode (adding a little tension to the body) is also habit forming. What's maintenance mode? Stand up. Stand up straight. Stand up when having office conversations. Walk and talk when you visit with friends. Practice putting on your shoes leaning against a wall instead of sitting down, which will also help your balance. Place a timer by your computer, and every 15 minutes, get up and do 5 jumping jacks, then resume sitting and computer time. Burning calories and practicing correct posture prolong your life. Thin people and people who move more, live longer.

Intellectual growth should commence at birth and cease only at death.

Albert Einstein

You live out the expectations that you choose to believe.

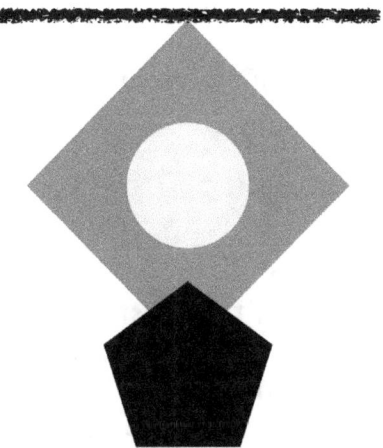

OODA Loop

OODA Loop.
Stands for...observe, orient, decide, act.
Observe your surroundings and where you fit in.
Orient yourself so you can best benefit.
Decide to take some action based on observing and orienting.
Act on your decision.
It works for business, relationships, aging, decision making, goal setting, and life.

Here's how it works for aging: you observe people who are aging well. They move well, they are alert, they have energy, they still like to do silly things like play on the monkey bars, and they engage in interesting conversations. That would be conversations that do not revolve solely around the doings of their grandchildren or their dogs.
Surprise. There is more to life than grandchildren and dogs.

Hang out with people who are aging well. They won't be dwelling on their age. That's orienting yourself by surrounding yourself with people you want to emulate, to be like them. That, instead of people who complain constantly and are searching for good nursing homes to live out their lives.

Decide that you will be someone who ages well.
Your brain believes anything that you tell it, so
tell it something that allows you to become the
person you would like to be.

Act on that decision. This is the tricky one.
People decide to do something all the time, but
fail to act on it. You must act to complete the
OODA loop. Stop that silly conversation in your
head that says you cannot do things because
you are getting old.

Keep repeating the OODA loop, adding more
information, making more choices.

You cannot do things you did as a child because,
well, you haven't practiced them in a while.
Get out there and try swinging from the monkey
bars. There is something to be said for silliness
that infects your whole being.

And allows you to stay young.

The difference between genius and stupidity is that genius has it's limits.

Wire Wrap For The Brain

Multiple Sclerosis is an autoimmune disease of the brain and spinal cord, and affects more than two million people worldwide. Half a million of those folks live in North America and Europe. You may know someone. You may be someone affected. If you are a woman, your chances of contracting MS are twice as good as a man.

We are not sure what causes MS, but we know what it is. And what it does. Immune cells collect in the upper spinal cord and brain, causing inflammation and the myelin sheath surrounding the nerves to degenerate. Big problem. It feels like limb weakness, fatigue, numbness and tingling, depression, vision issues, slurred speech, and memory difficulties. But not all the time. The symptoms come and go, which makes it frustrating. They never appear when you go to the doctor complaining about them.

What to do? Build up that myelin sheath to help protect your nerves.

Myelin is a protective wrap around the nerves. Think of electrical tape around wires. We know, from neuroscience, how to build the myelin sheath. It's deep, deliberate practice. That would be practice wherein you actually pay attention to what you are doing, not mindlessly running on a NordicTrack, or swimming endless laps in an effort to improve skill, all the while with your brain in neutral. The more deep, conscious practice, the more myelin is formed and the bigger the wrap around the nerves. This is protection from disease, drugs, stress, poor life habits, and those pesky immune cells. Try learning a new skill. That too forms myelin. Deep, deliberate practice is practicing with the expectation that you will get better, staying in the moment of practice and not wandering away mentally, analyzing any errors, visualizing the skill, and repeating the process. Fail forward. Deep practice takes concentration and repetition. Practice, make errors, analyze, slow down, practice some more. Wrap your nerves with myelin and protect your brain from autoimmune diseases. I could be wrong about this, but what if I'm not?

Many of life's failures are people
who did not realize how close

they were to success

when they gave up.

Thomas Edison

We are not in this

to

test the waters,

we are in this

to

make waves.

Dempsey Dybdahl

Appreciation

A decision is a judgement.

It is a choice between alternatives.

It is rarely a choice between right and wrong.

It is at best a choice between "almost right" and "probably wrong."

Dempsey Dybdahl

What's With The Weather?

Summer is making an appearance early this year in Seattle with blue skies and warm weather. I have been outside more than to just collect mail and run to my car, parked 20 feet away.

I am affected by sunlight and gray days. When it's dark, dreary, and frigid in the winter, I suffer. Don't open the drapes; it's too gray outside. Stay in and turn the lights on, I shelter myself from the cold. The drizzle of rain is soothing, gray skies are not. I get cranky, depressed, moody, and eat the wrong things: sugar laden, fat filled comfort foods. This is me waiting for summer, and warmth. Perhaps I'm a lizard, searching for a warm rock. Phoenix in August is heaven to me.

When we feel out-of-sorts and can't explain why, it might be that an external force is affecting us, like weather: hurricane, tornado, hot spell, cold blustery afternoon. Or maybe it's toxic relationships, too much food, lack of sleep, more anxiety than is healthy, or not enough movement throughout the day. A body at rest.......stays there. It settles. Everything affects everything else, including mood. With awareness comes the ability to recognize that something isn't working, and the ability to change it. Anything can affect anything else. Do something different to reengage your brain and your energy.

Variations of workouts come to me more in the winter than the summer. Imagination surfaces in cold weather, and I have more curiosity. I have to keep moving to stay warm and keep my mind engaged. It's a productive time, the damp and dreary. But I don't have to like the weather.

When it's warm, I go outside and savor the sunlight, thinking nothing thoughts. Everything in time: Spring, Summer, Winter, Fall; even the seasons know that change is healthy. Life is change. Accept it, embrace it, use it.

We can let circumstances rule us, or we can take charge and rule our lives from within.

Earl Nightingale

If you work, it will lead to
something.

It's the people who do

all of the work

all of the time

who eventually catch on

to things.

How Paying Attention Helps Recovery

Stupid shoes caused a fall. The shoes encased my foot and it couldn't move, couldn't feel the ground. My brain had no idea what kind of surface, slippery or bumpy, was under my feet, and I fell. Turned out, I nicked my lateral meniscus on my left knee, and needed surgery. That was four years ago.

I was training to become a trainer with Z-Health (zhealth.net), a company that marries neuroscience with movement by teaching the body better communication with it's nervous system and brain. Recovery went well; my knee is fine.

I injured my other knee at the same time, but it took awhile to complain. For the last year, kneeling caused sharp pain. I returned to the same surgeon, for surgery on the other knee. As soon as I was scheduled for surgery, I began strengthening quads, hips, and knee ligaments. Upped my cardio. Added eye drills and balance work. I needed balance after surgery and I wanted the recovery process minimal. I rested well, and cut out as much sugar as I could stand. This, in an effort to be in the best possible shape for an assault on my knee. I have been through this before, I know the rehab procedures. Light eating, breath work, eye drills, balance work, and joint mobility have speeded up recovery.

Day 5; I have no pain, I walk up and down stairs without hitching a hip, my swelling is subsiding, and I do drills every day, several times. Healing is a process that done well, is a mild annoyance, not future and permanent incapacitation. Life is dings, I know rehab.

I expect to be as good as new when healed. I am not 17 anymore; it takes time, probably a couple of years to be completely healed on the inside, although it may feel fine on the outside in a couple of months. Now I am strengthening quads again, and still doing the eye drills and the balance work. If you think that a couple of years is too much work, then get ready for continued issues, and lack of choice. For me, this is a cheap price to pay for life without pain, without medication, without wheelchairs and walkers, without giving up the life to which I have become accustomed, without remorse.

Because I saw surgery as a battle, I prepared holistically, involving diet, rest, breath work, joint mobility, visual and vestibular input. The body is a whole. Recovery should be whole. I had a great team surrounding the process of surgery and rehab. The whole body participating in whole recovery. Aging well isn't for everyone. You have to work at it. For my money, it's the only choice.

Actions speak louder than words but not nearly as often.

Mark Twain

Life is either

a daring adventure

or

nothing at all.

Helen Keller

Why Numbers Matter

3 891 **73**28**8** 56356**29** 4 **3492**
37 **2**9446 2 **56** 655 **3589**

My dad was 67 years old when he died. He was way too young. But he had issues: gout, high blood pressure, high cholesterol, diabetes. He had a stroke 8 years before his death, was 60 pounds overweight for the last 30 years of his life, and had not exercised since he was in boot camp in the Army 45 years before.

My daughter was 5 years old at the time.

What this means is that he was deprived of watching his first granddaughter grow up, and she never knew him.

If this isn't a reason for paying attention to our aging process, I don't know what is.

There is a remedy for everything.....

it is called

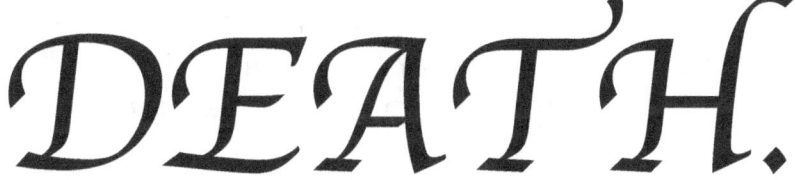

DEATH.

Portuguese proverb

When I Die

A life well lived should contain some fear along the way, but no regrets. Regret means that I didn't quite get the concept of acceptance of myself, and let fear dominate my life. I don't "have to" have some risk and novelty and interest in my life. I am not forced to do anything. I choose to. Every day I make that choice.

Maybe we feel that we don't have enough information to make good decisions. No fool would jump out of an airplane without a parachute. But given one, and instruction, and practice at lower elevations, we might jump out of that plane, were we inclined. If we have a parachute, instruction and practice, and want to jump and still don't, the consequence will be regret. Which is a loose translation of: what could have been.

If we fear looking stupid, if no one we know has done this whatever thing it is that we want to do, if we are going to have to go it alone, if everyone says we're crazy to start a new business, learn a foreign language at our age (whatever that is), or take up line dancing………..if we give in to that thinking, we will have regrets. What might have been. That business may succeed wildly, we may travel to that foreign country, we may move more because of line dancing, thus insuring aging mobility. And we might have had a great time trying something new. Laughing out loud great time.

When I die, I want to be used up. I want to look slightly ragged, clothes askew, like I have had an interesting and eventful life. I want to slide into my grave with one shoe off, missing some lipstick, and hear someone say, "There was a life well lived."

The end of life is death, not disease. The end of disease is regret.

life

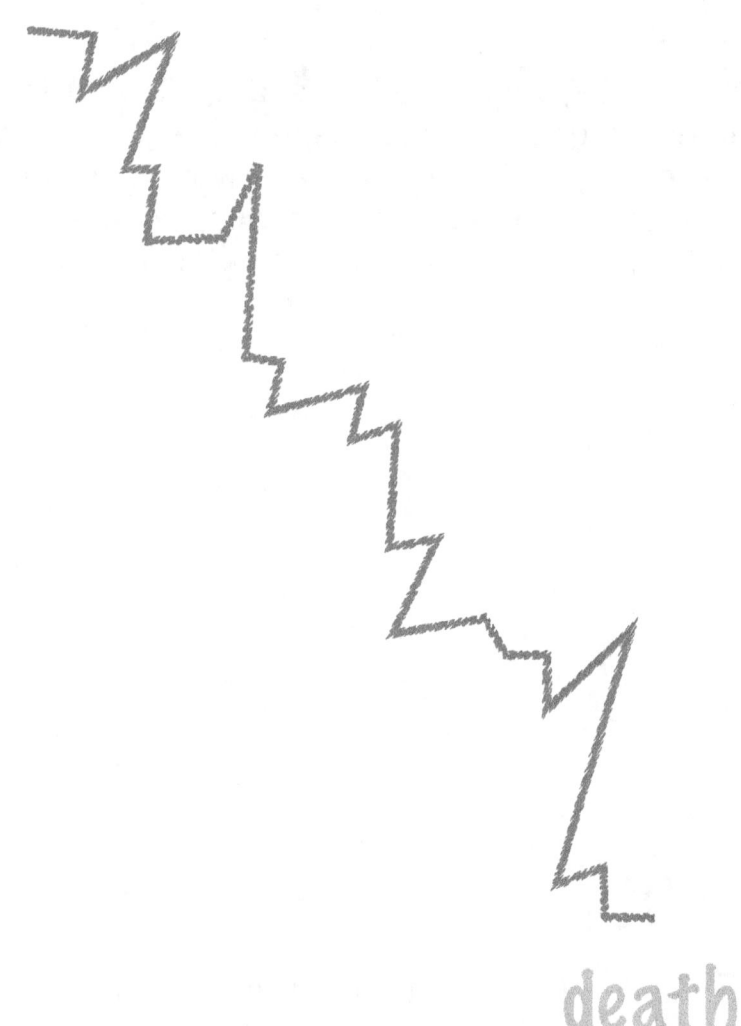

death

What if the hokey pokey

is

what it's all about?

This ending is intended to be a beginning for Aging Intelligently.

Use your brain

Move your body

With thanks:

to my clients, who give me great ideas,

my husband, Eric, who applauds my efforts

and Jen Waak, who wrestled this into production.

You can reach Dempsey at
www.Queendempsey@gmail.com.

Or, to see what's new, visit
www.DempseysMobilityJoint.com/blog

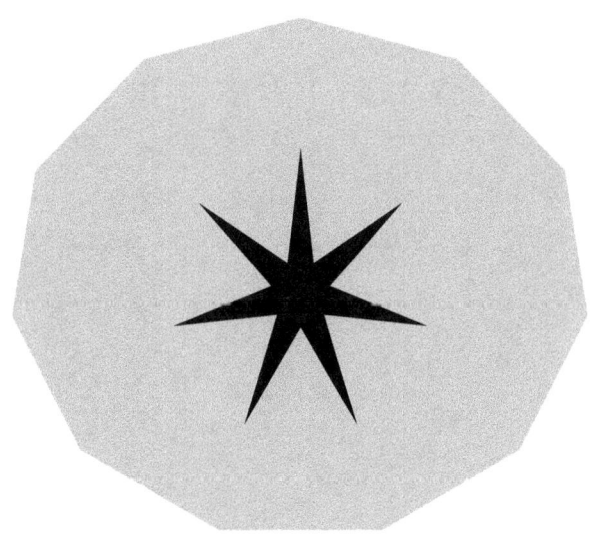

Dempsey Dybdahl

www.ingramcontent.com/pod-product-compliance
Lightning Source LLC
Chambersburg PA
CBHW070208290526

45789CB00002B/945